I0435797

21 Superfoods for the Elderly

The Top 21 Superfoods in Every Elderly Diet to Keep Them Healthy and Strong

Sarah Sparrow

PUBLISHED BY:
Sarah Sparrow
Copyright © 2012

Disclaimer

The information contained in this book is for general information purposes only. The information is provided by the authors and while we endeavor to keep the information up to date and correct, we make no representations or warranties of any kind, express or implied, about the completeness, accuracy, reliability, suitability or availability with respect to the book or the information, products, services, or related graphics contained in the book for any purpose. Any reliance you place on such information is therefore strictly at your own risk.

Table of Contents

Chapter 1: Introduction

The Definition of Superfoods

The word "superfoods" is not a scientific term. Nutrition scientists as well as licensed dieticians don't recognize this word as a norm in the field of science. However, "superfood" is commonly used in marketing agendas. And the term is now widely accepted by health enthusiasts all over the world.

When one hears the word superfood, food groups that are high in vitamins, minerals, phytonutrients, and antioxidants quickly come to mind. These foods are high in fiber content, and have typically low amount of calories. While there may be instances when food sources may carry some form of saturated fat and artificial ingredients, only a minimal amount of these negative properties are present in the food products.

Superfoods are recommended for everyone, as we all need to eat foods that are high in nutrition in order to have a healthy body. The elderly will also particularly benefit from these types of food as their condition can be very fragile and weak. Regular consumption of foods that are considered to be "super" can therefore improve their overall standing and well-being.

Preparing and Choosing Superfoods for the Elderly

The elderly are particularly choosy with the types of food that they eat. As their sense of smell and taste starts to deteriorate, their appetite for eating tends to decline too. Their caretakers should therefore be able to provide them with foods that are not only tasty, but nutritious as well.

The types of food that are served to elderly people should be loaded with natural vitamins and minerals as well as live enzymes. And as they are prone to having bowel irregularity, high-fiber foods should also be included in their diet. The amount of calories taken in daily should also be monitored closely as gaining weight can be quite risky for people over 60. With all the illnesses related to aging, serious complications like obesity and diabetes may arise when one gains too much weight.

Fruits and vegetables are always the best sources for vitamins and minerals. Fruits and veggies that can be classified as "superfoods" have bright colors, so you can take that as a cue as to their nutritional value.

How to Prepare Superfoods When Served to the Elderly

As much as possible, fruits and vegetables should be served in their raw form as they are more nutritious that way. However, as majority of the elderly already have chewing problems, the food's overall texture and digestibility also need to be considered.

Lean meat, poultry, and fish are all good sources of protein. And any of these varieties can be given to the elderly in one serving portion per meal. Fruits and veggies can then be served as side dishes or appetizers.

Green salad is particularly good for digestion as the ingredients in this type of recipe carry high doses of fiber. Aside from helping in digestion, dietary fiber also aids in promoting regular bowel movement.

If you are going to serve soup, come up with a recipe that will result in a clear but tasty dish. This is way better than cream-type of soups as the creamer contains high amounts of calories. Onion soup is particularly beneficial to individuals in their senior years, and you can add in other veggies to the mixture to make it more delicious.

Make it a point, too, that brown rice is served to the elderly instead of white rice. Aside from being more nutritious, brown rice is also easier to digest.

How to Superfood the Elderly's Diet Plan

If you think that preparing a superfood meal can be expensive and troublesome, then think again. Superfood recipes are actually easy to create, and the ingredients are really quite cheap too.

If you purchase fruits and vegetables that are in season, you can make smoothie recipes as well as different types of soups, salads and casseroles. Just make sure that you only buy a small amount of produce at a time as getting these in bulk can only result in spoiled and rotten food if these are not consumed immediately.

Aside from fruits and veggies, you can also incorporate oatmeal, eggs, and tea drinks when serving food to an aging person. Meat products should also be included in main meals as long as these are lean and tender.

Listed below are some of the basic ingredients that you can use in superfood recipes for the elderly.

- **Kale** – This vegetable is very affordable as a cup of kale leaves will only cost you around 60 cents. It can be included in different types of recipes to increase its nutritional value and it won't ruin the taste of dishes.

  This is a popular superfood as it contains high amounts of vitamins (A, B, C and E) and minerals (iron, manganese, zinc, etc) as well as antioxidants. It can therefore boost the immune system of the elderly.

- **Broccoli** – For just about a dollar per serving, this veggie can provide aging people with calcium in order to promote bone health. Its vitamins A and C properties are also anti-cancer, so it can help the system to resist such diseases.

  Broccoli can be served raw (as an ingredient in juice recipes), steamed, or stir fried. This veggie also makes a good addition in pasta and soup dishes as it adds a distinct taste to the meal.

- **Sweet Potatoes** – A serving of sweet potatoes only costs around 43 cents, and yet its nutritional value is extremely high. The B vitamins contained in this root crop is essential for cellular health, and its beta carotene contents is an anti-cancer agent. Since it is also loaded with vitamin A that's especially good for the skin, the development of wrinkles and lines can be controlled and avoided.

  This is a versatile veggie, so you can use it as an ingredient in soups and casseroles. Potatoes are also delicious when baked or mashed; and they can replace a rice meal.

- **Blueberries** – This type of berry is extremely cheap especially when in season, so be sure to take advantage of its low price whenever you can. Because of its delicious taste, it can be eaten fresh as it is. You can also include it in smoothie recipes or add a few pieces in cereals and oatmeal mixture.

  The high antioxidant content of blueberries enables the body of the elderly to adapt to the aging process more efficiently. Their bodies become more resistant to illnesses and their overall stress levels are also kept to a minimum.

- **Eggs** – An egg will only cost you about 20 cents per piece. While its cholesterol content is quite high, it can be very beneficial to the body when taken in moderation.

  Eggs are a good source of protein, which can provide the elderly with the needed energy so as not to feel weak and lethargic. And it also has Choline which aids in brain health so that individuals in their senior years don't become prone to Alzheimer's disease.

- **Oatmeal** – Oatmeal is very easy to prepare and you can even add other nutritional foods in it to make it a "super superfood" (cinnamon, fruits, nuts, raisins, etc.). Because of its high fiber component, the body will not suffer from constipation problems.

  Oatmeal is also fortified with iron, zinc, and manganese; and all of these minerals promote healthy blood and bones. Its antioxidant properties also help in reducing the risk of developing inflammations and infections inside the body.

- **Tea** – As there's a wide variety of teas out on the market today, you will find that there are cheap as well as expensive teas. If you want to economize and yet reap the nutritional value of this type of superfood, you can simply get the regular flavored green tea or black tea. The flavored variety can indeed be very expensive, but you can add honey or lemon to regular teas to make them more delicious and enjoyable.

The green and black tea varieties are considered to be particularly good for the elderly. They will benefit from its high antioxidant properties to enhance their immune system, and teas have calming and soothing effects too.

The Superfood Swap

As you would really want to increase the nutritional value of the elderly's food consumption, you should think of clever ways to replace regular meals with healthier ones. One way of doing this is to replace a low-nutrition type of food with a superfood diet as much as you can.

For example, if you are going to serve tacos for snack, you can make use of black beans as the main ingredient instead of beef. Beans are high in fiber and protein, and they are very affordable too.

Because of its starch contents, white potatoes are seldom served to the elderly. Sweet potatoes are more suitable to their condition, as this is low in starch yet high in fiber and vitamins.

Milk shakes which can be very high in calories can be replaced with smoothies, which are just as tasty and refreshing. You can also create juice diet recipes using fruit and vegetable ingredients.

Even potato chips can be replaced with more nutritional alternatives. Kale chips and spinach chips can be enjoyed by the elderly as snacks when presented and served creatively.

Chapter 2: The Elderly Nutrition

The nutritional needs of people change as they get older. People who are over 60 years old need a particular type of diet as their activities and bodily functions are no longer as demanding as it was years ago. Special precautionary measures should also be taken as the condition of the elderly can be very sensitive.

Essential Nutrients that Should Be Included in the Diet of the Elderly

There are no exact diet plans for the elderly as their conditions vary from one another. It will therefore depend on a particular individual's present state of health as well as overall situation.

Vitamins and Minerals

Foods that are loaded with nutrients should also be included in their regular meals as these will make their bodies strong and resistant to diseases. That's why a wide variety of dishes should be in their daily menu so that they will not lose their appetite. Fruits and vegetables that carry high amounts of vitamins and minerals are particularly recommended to the elderly, while those that have high calorie contents should be avoided. This way, they can get their regular dose of vitamins A, B, C and E from natural food sources.

Protein

Those who are generally fit need a good dose of energy food so that they can cope with their daily activities better. Protein food should also be made available to them as this will aid in keeping their muscles strong.

Iron

The older one gets, the higher is the need for iron. This mineral can correct anemic conditions which can be prevalent to the elderly. You can serve them green leafy vegetables in soup or salad form so as to provide them with a good source of iron.

Zinc

This mineral is needed if you want a healthy and strong immune system. And it's very helpful to the elderly as it helps in healing wounds both inside and outside the body. That's why it can even improve the condition of ulcers, as these are little wounds inside the linings of the intestines.

Whole meal breads and shellfish are some of the best sources of zinc. But this mineral can be found in most vegetables too.

Calcium

Bone health is very important to old people as their bones become more and more fragile through the years. Calcium strengthens the bones, and it will lower the risk of developing osteoporosis and other forms of bone degeneration.

Milk and other dairy products are good sources of calcium too. However, only low-fat milk is recommended as regular milk contains high amounts of calories.

Vitamin D

The body needs vitamin D in order for the calcium to be absorbed properly. You can serve the elderly sardines, eggs, and butter, but these only carry a minimal amount of said vitamin.

The best source of vitamin D is exposure to the sun. Morning sun is particularly beneficial, and the best time to do this is around 7AM to 8AM.

Vitamin C

The C vitamin is extremely important in all stages of one's life as it's a natural immune booster. It makes the body resistant to diseases, and it also allows for quick recovery when one is suffering from an illness. This is also an antioxidant, so it helps in battling free radicals that can lead to cancer as well.

Fiber

High fiber foods are recommended to the elderly, so be sure to include oatmeal and cereal meals to their daily regimen. These types of food will stimulate the digestive system to function properly so as to avoid constipation problems.

Fluid

Old people are particularly at risk of dehydration because their kidneys are no longer as efficient as they used to be. Furthermore, at this stage in one's life, the thirst sensation has already tremendously decreased.

If you are taking care of a loved one or a patient, it may be necessary to persuade them to drink frequently. Otherwise, they may altogether forget that they still need to drink some form of liquid even if they don't feel thirsty.

Although water is enough, old folks may be more encouraged to drink fresh juices; so always make these types of drinks available to them too. You can even mix fruits and vegetables in one drink so as to make it more powerful and potent.

A Variation in Diet

A varied diet is most beneficial to the elderly as their appetites tend to decline with age. The foods that are served to them should therefore be as appealing as they are tasty, and variation is an important factor too.

Their meals and snacks should always be nutritious and easy to swallow. And as their fluid intake is particularly important, water, fruit juices and herbal teas should be made available to them at all times.

Health Benefits of Superfoods to the Elderly

Consuming superfoods is beneficial to the elderly because it can improve their overall health condition. Listed below are some of the good effects that can be derived from eating a healthy diet.

- To Prevent Illnesses – As the body's immune system is strengthened, it becomes more resistant to germs, bacteria and viruses.

- For Brain Health – Having sufficient nutrients will enable the body to bring a proper supply of oxygen to the brain. This helps improve memory, and diseases like Alzheimer's disease and dementia can also be avoided.

- To Gain Energy – Old people tend to feel weak and lethargic because their internal organs are no longer as efficient as they used to be. However, by supplying these organs with natural sources of vitamins and minerals, they can be stimulated to function normally so that nourishment from food can be distributed well inside the body.

- Anti-Aging – Superfoods are said to delay the signs of aging. Their antioxidant properties not only strengthen the body from inside, but one's overall look can also be enhanced. Vitamins A and C are also very helpful in keeping the skin elastic, so development of lines and wrinkles particularly on the face area can also be avoided or delayed.

- Natural Pain Reliever – There are certain vitamins and minerals (Potassium, B Vitamins, etc.) that help reduce joint pains. Symptoms of rheumatism can therefore improve through proper diet and nourishment.

- Bone Health – Superfoods contain calcium which is essential for bone and teeth health. The elderly need this mineral as they are prone to osteoporosis and chewing problems.

- Eye Health – Old people lose their vision in the passage of time. That's why it's important that their diet is high in Vitamin A and lutein so as to assist their vision health. These components also aid in avoiding the development of cataracts, glaucoma, and macular degeneration.

- Heart Health – The omega 3 composition contained in superfoods is particularly good for the heart. This makes the elderly less prone to strokes and heart attacks.

- Proper Digestion – Superfoods generally carry high levels of dietary fiber. This aids in natural detoxification of the body, and it also relieves symptoms of constipation and irregular bowel movement.

- Cellular Health – The antioxidant properties of superfood enable the body to become resistant to free radicals. The growth of tumors can therefore be hindered, and cancer cells can even be killed.

How Many Calories per Day is Suggested to the Elderly?

The recommended daily calorie intake for the elderly will depend on the person's gender and actual age. For 50 to 70 year-old male, one may take around 2,299 calories in a day. As for females in the same age bracket, only about 1,980 calories per day is advised.

For males aging 70 and up, a maximum of 2,050 calories per day is allowed. For the female elderly, only around 1,870 calories per day is recommended.

As you can see, the recommended daily calorie intake decreases as one gets older and older. The reason behind this is that old people no longer need too much calories in their old age as their bodies cannot burn these anymore. Moreover, high calorie intake can result in gaining a lot of weight, which in turn can lead to complications.

Those who are taking care of elderly parents, relatives, or patients should therefore monitor the amount of calories consumed by a person in his or her senior years very closely. Protein foods like meat can indeed help in maintaining muscle mass, but only around 10% to 35 % of the total dietary requirement should be comprised of this food group as it is one of the main sources of calories.

Carbohydrates, on the other hand, can be consumed anywhere from 45% to 65% as this is a source of energy. Foods that are rich in carbohydrates include rice and pasta, so caretakers of the elderly should also monitor these so as not to go beyond the allowed proportions.

Fatty foods like chocolates should be avoided as much as possible, and can just be given as treats. While it can contribute to building body mass, it can cause tooth decay and loss of appetite. Only around 20% of the total food intake can be comprised of fatty foods like this.

In order to balance out the negative effects of some of the sources of fat and calories, meals should be integrated with high fiber sources. Fruits and vegetables are particularly recommended as these are easy to digest and nutritious as well. Moreover, dietary fiber aids in proper digestion and regular bowel movement.

Why Malnutrition is a Critical Health Issue Among Elder People

People in their 50s, 60s, 70s, and up have different nutritional requirements than people who are younger. At this stage, their activities have already changed and lightened up. That's why eating meals in the wrong proportions can be harmful to their general condition as they may be lacking in some nutrients and over-supplied with elements that are actually harmful to their condition.

An unbalanced diet can be dangerous for the elderly as it can lead to a lot of complications and health problems. As the body is not fully nourished, it can be prone to liver and kidney diseases and even result in cancer.

A weak immune system is also prone to lung diseases like pneumonia and tuberculosis. While TB can be cured, it still requires a long and tedious process. And pneumonia can be very deadly if not treated properly.

Poor nutrition can also result in mental impairment due to iodine deficiency. An elderly person therefore becomes more prone to depression and anxiety, and they can show symptoms of Obsessive Compulsive Disorder (OCD). Dementia, bipolar syndrome, and schizophrenia can also arise from malnutrition.

In order to avoid malnutrition in the elderly, you can look at the underlying issue behind the problem. Find out the reason why a person loses his or her appetite. Is it because of the general presentation of the food? Or is it because of the snacks that have been consumed before the main meals? Perhaps there are chewing or swallowing problems that you are not aware of? Ask the individual person directly so as to find out about the problem; and seek for an effective solution.

Tips to Avoid Malnutrition

Here are 16 tips to help you take care of an elderly and avoid malnutrition.

Always provide them with healthy foods and snacks

Make it a point that they get their carbohydrates from healthy sources like brown rice and whole meal bread.

The same goes for their protein requirements; so it's better to serve them meat from poultry and fish products rather than red meat.

As for their snacks, you can entice them with fruits. Apples, oranges, bananas, grapes, pears, strawberries, and cherries are all filled with vitamins and minerals, and they are extremely delicious too. Cakes and pastries should only be given occasionally as these are high in sugar.

Use fresh herbs to flavor their food

Fresh ingredients are always better than unnatural products. You can use basil, thyme, rosemary, cilantro, and parsley to add flavor to dishes. These types of herbs also provide meals with a delicious and appealing scent.

Use pre-packed supplements once in a while

It may be necessary for the really picky eaters to consume supplemental products that are fortified with vitamins and minerals. Protein shakes and other nutritional beverages can be purchased and served to the elderly to aid in their nutrition.

Promote exercise

Aside from resulting in having stronger bones and muscles, regular exercise can also stimulate one's appetite. You should therefore encourage the elderly to walk around 30 minutes to 1 hour before a meal.

Arrange for Social Activities

Encourage old people to socialize with others by arranging parties and other forms of get-together activities. You can then serve healthy meals during the occasion so as to encourage them to eat a healthy diet while socializing with friends.

Serve a wide variety of food

Variety in the weekly menu is a must if you want to keep their appetite going. Make sure that the meals are flavorful and not spicy, and that the presentation is appealing to the eyes as well.

Monitor the regularity of meals

As the digestive system of the elderly is no longer as functional as it used to be, they should only be served small meals at a time. At this point in their lives, small frequent meals are more advisable than 3 big meals in a day.

Check the nutritional density of food

Old people tend to lose their appetites quickly once their stomachs are full. The one in charge of their meals should therefore make it a point that nutritious meals are served first before less nutritious types of food. Low nutrient types of beverages, for example (tea and coffee), can be filling. So these shouldn't be served before meals as they can lose their appetite and refuse to eat.

Serve them energy food

You can give them protein-rich foods like milk, cheese, and yogurt to increase their energy. These types of food are also rich in calcium, so it also helps in maintaining healthy bones and teeth.

Check for dental problems

Should the elderly under your care be suffering from teeth problems, you should take them to the dentist right away. Furthermore, they should only be served with soft-textured meals so as to encourage them to eat.

If you are going to prepare meat recipes, you can chop the meat into small pieces so that these are easier to chew. Or better yet, you can mince them and add sauces to make them moist and tender. And if you are going to serve them bread, remove the crust as it can be too hard for them to chew.

Monitor their fluid intake

Old people rarely feel thirsty anymore as their activities are already limited. However, proper hydration is still important as it is the basis for one's overall health. The elderly should always be encouraged to drink water, and you can also add variety to their drinks by serving them fresh juices.

Check their alcohol intake

Too much alcohol can be harmful to old people as they can easily get dehydrated. And alcohol depletes the body of water. While a glass of wine has many health benefits, this should be consumed in moderation (about one glass a day is enough).

Prepare their food preferences

Do give in to the elderly's request when they ask for certain meals and food recipes. As long as these are prepared using healthy ingredients, it will not harm them. On the contrary, you might even notice that their appetites are stimulated when served with their favorite dishes.

Give them enough time to eat

You shouldn't hurry them up while eating as some people are just naturally slow eaters. Allow them to enjoy their meal, without the pressure of time constraints. And don't reprimand them for eating too slow as they can easily lose their appetite when scolded.

Use multivitamin supplements

Multivitamin supplements can be given to old people who are not eating well. This will ensure that they are getting the minimum daily requirements of vitamins and minerals that their body need.

Provide for a pleasant ambiance

Meals become more enjoyable when shared with friends and relatives. If you are taking care of a loved one, be sure to eat with them during meals. This will lift their spirits up and increase their appetite.

Chapter 3: Top Foods to Avoid

There are foods that are good for the elderly, and there are also those that are bad. By knowing which types of foods to avoid will help in keeping them healthy and problem-free.

Deep-Fried Food

Greasy foods are hard to digest, and these can cause stomach problems among the elderly. The calories contained in oily products are also particularly high, so this can also lead to obesity if an individual's metabolism is very slow. Too much saturated fat in the diet can even cause brain problems as it can hinder the proper circulation of oxygen. And one of the deadliest complications of too much grease in one's diet is the development of cancer.

Grilled Meals

As delicious as grilled meals may be, these are not good for the health. Old people are especially vulnerable to diseases as they already have a weak immune system. The smoke in grilling foods contains carcinogenic materials, and this poses the risk of having cancer.

Processed Foods

It's convenient to eat and serve processed foods, but these contain preservatives and additives to help them stay fresh for an extended period of time. While these types of food may taste really good because of artificial flavoring, they carry very minimal doses of vitamins and minerals. And since they are loaded with artificial ingredients, they can cause stomach problems like diarrhea, constipation, and even colon cancer.

Cold Drinks

It's quite alright for the elderly to consume cold drinks once in a while. However, they should not get into the habit of always drinking icy drinks as this can hinder the production of live enzymes in the digestive system. And as we all know, these enzymes are needed for proper digestion.

Sweet Stuff

The sugar contents of pastries, cakes, cookies, candies, and chocolates can disturb the blood sugar levels of old people easily. While you can give these types of treats moderately, it can be very dangerous if they consume too much of it. An abrupt increase in sugar levels can cause problems like stroke and heart attack. And too much sugar can also lead to hypertension and diabetes.

Animal Intestines

Animal internal organs contain high amounts of fat and cholesterol. These should not be included in the regular diet of old people as they can trigger heart attacks and strokes.

Animal Blood

Recipes that call for the use of animal blood should also be avoided as blood is also high in cholesterol. Those with existing heart problems can suffer from hypertension and cardiac arrest which can be life-threatening. Even those without heart problems should not be served with these types of recipes as old people are simply prone to developing heart problems when their cholesterol levels are not kept at the right balance.

Convenience Food

Some examples of food that are made for convenience include instant noodles and canned goods. These are very easy to prepare, but they have no nutritional value at all. In fact, these types of foods are loaded with preservatives and coloring, so they may even cause cancer in the long run.

Expired Food

Old people have the habit of eating expired food, which is a really bad practice. Their caretakers should discourage them from doing this as eating spoiled food can lead to an upset stomach. Or worse, one may even suffer from food poisoning.

Chapter 4: Overcoming Obstacles to Eating Healthy Food

There are a lot of reasons why old people have eating problems. Below you will find some of the most common obstacles that are faced by the elderly in eating healthy.

Eating Alone

When one is left alone, as when a husband or wife dies, the remaining individual is faced with the challenge of eating alone. This can lead to depression as the loved one is remembered every time one sits at the dinner table to have a meal. The sadness can be particularly felt if the dearly departed is the one in charge of cooking as the one left will miss the homemade recipes usually served to him or her.

Preparing a meal for one person is also not as enjoyable as preparing for two. And even if one gets past the preparation stage, eating alone is simply not looked forward to. In this case, it may be necessary to share meals with an elderly who just lost a spouse so as to help him or her get past the sadness stage.

Loss of Appetite

There are many reasons why an aging person can lose the appetite for eating. Because of hormonal imbalance, one may have good appetite today and experience loss of appetite the next day. This is quite normal for old people; so the best thing to do is to serve them small meals at a time instead of forcing them to eat 3 big meals in a day. You can also entice them to eat by serving them their favorite dishes on those days when they don't have the appetite to eat.

Loss of appetite can also be attributed to their deteriorating state of mind. An old person's brain is not as functional as it used to be, so even the sense of taste and smell are also affected. The sense of sight also sends signals to the brain, so it would also help if the food served to them have a pleasing appearance.

The decline in one's regular activities can also lead to loss of appetite as the body has fewer requirements for energy foods. For this reason, old people should be encouraged to perform even mild forms of exercises like walking and stretching to increase one's appetite.

Although it can be quite normal for the elderly to lose their appetite once in a while, the situation shouldn't be taken lightly. Loss of appetite can be a symptom of more serious diseases, so it may be necessary to consult a doctor if the condition is worsening. Problems of the heart, kidneys, liver, and lungs can manifest in the form of depression and loss of appetite.

And if an elderly is under medication and is taking a lot of prescription drugs, it can also be one of the many side effects of the medicine. This should be reported to the doctor so as to find a remedy for the problem.

Dry Mouth

Having dry mouth is common to the elderly as they are drinking less and less fluids. As one gets along in years, the ability to detect thirst is hampered. Because of this, the secretion of saliva is also affected and swallowing food becomes a tedious task.

In order to help them chew and swallow the foods that are served to them, these should be served with sauces and dips. Fish meals should be soft, and meat dishes should be very tender and moist.

You can also serve them with easy to swallow food like oatmeal instead of hard cereals that they can choke on. Soups, broths, and fresh juices can also accompany their meals.

Rough grain food products like rice and grain can also be replaced with mashed potatoes. Potatoes are heavy on the stomach just like rice, and they're very nutritious too. In fact, potatoes can even assist in maintaining muscle mass.

If you are going to give them vegetables, these are best served steamed so as to retain their nutritional value. However, some produce are quite tough, so it may be more practical to puree them and serve them as liquid meals. This way, they're easier to swallow and more easily digestible too.

There are simple solutions to ease the condition of having dry mouths among the elderly. Encouraging them to drink at least 8 glasses of water every day will stimulate the production of saliva. You can also give them candies once in a while, as these can stimulate the salivary glands to produce saliva.

Difficulty in Chewing

Ill-fitting dentures as well as tooth problems can hinder a person from eating well. It can be painful to chew on hard types of food, so the elderly may simply choose not to eat. A dentist should be consulted right away so that any dental and oral problems can be treated immediately.

As old people are really prone to dental problems, they should only be served with soft meals. Meat products should be cooked really well so that they can be chewed and digested properly.

As even fruits and vegetables may seem too tough for those with tooth and gum problems, it may be necessary to process these in the juicer or blender. You can even combine fruits and vegetables in one powerful juice drink as long as the taste can be tolerated well.

Chapter 5: Introduction to the 21 Superfoods for the Elderly

As the nutrients present in superfoods can help sustain the health of the elderly, it's important to focus on the types of food that fall under this category. In the next 7 chapters, you will be presented with the 21 types of superfoods that are especially beneficial to the elderly diet. They are segregated into 7 sections to represent those foods that are categorized as fatty fish, nuts, vegetables, fruits, dairy, grain and healthy beverages. The nutritional benefits of the different types of food under each group are also discussed briefly so as to serve as a guide to the elderly themselves or to their caretakers.

Chapter 6: Fatty Fish

Fatty Fish is considered to be a superfood because it contains Omega 3, protein, Vitamin D and Vitamin B12. Both Salmon and tuna fall under this category, so both types of fish are advised to be included in the dietary plans of the elderly.

Salmon

You have the option of removing the skin on the salmon before cooking as it can be contaminated with chemicals and other forms of pollutants in the water. This type of fish cooks easily, so you need to monitor it closely to avoid overcooking. When cooked just right, this is a delicious meal to have, and even adults in their senior years will enjoy it. The fish meat tastes really good, and it's moist and tender as well. The best types of salmon recipes involve steaming, baking and broiling.

The Omega 3 components found in salmon help in keeping the heart healthy. It is also good for the brain, so that the elderly will be less prone to Alzheimer's disease, dementia, and other similar forms of mental illness. Its B12 properties make the system more secure as it helps in controlling inflammations and infections. Even the insulin levels of those who are suffering from diabetes can be effectively maintained so as to avoid complications.

Tuna

Tuna fish is high in Omega 3, protein, magnesium, selenium, potassium, and B vitamins. Its Omega 3 content can make the heart stronger, and it also promotes regular heartbeat.

This type of fish also carries detoxifying agents, so even the liver can be cleansed of stored drugs, pesticides, and heavy metals that may have accumulated through the years.

The antioxidant properties contain in tuna can also help the elderly avoid cancer problems. The ovaries, digestive tract, pancreas, mouth, esophagus, kidneys and colon will all be more resistant to diseases.

Benefits of Omega 3 Fish Oil from Fatty Fish

Fatty fish oil should be included in the elderly diet because it will make them healthier. They will be less prone to diseases and pains that are associated with growing old, so that they can live happier and longer lives.

Improve Eye Health

As one gets older, the eyesight begins to decline. This can be attributed to the weakening of eye muscles and tissues which enable a person to see clearly. By taking fish oil, further degeneration of eye health can be prevented. Symptoms of cataracts, glaucoma, and macular degeneration can be delayed for years.

Maintain Brain Functions

Omega 3 benefits the brain as it prevents the inflammation of cells on this part of the body. A person's cognitive ability can therefore be preserved, and diseases like dementia and Alzheimer's disease can also be prevented.

Reduce Joint Pain

The fatty fish oil can also serve as a lubricant for the joints. This will therefore reduce the pain of arthritis and rheumatism which are both associated with aging.

Cancer-Fighting

The Omega 3 components of fatty fish like tuna and salmon can stop the growth of cancer cells. In fact, regular intake of this nutritious oil can even kill cancer cells.

For Heart Health

The healthy oil contained in fatty fish can increase a person's good cholesterol while decreasing the bad cholesterol simultaneously. The heart's veins and arteries are also strengthened so as to avoid deadly heart diseases like stroke and cardiac arrest.

How Much Fatty Fish Can Be Served to the Elderly?

As the Omega 3 component is particularly helpful to the mind health of old people, this can be served in large doses. 3 or more servings in a week can provide the best results as other essential nutrients are present in this type of food as well. However, as the appetite of old folks can sometimes diminish unexpectedly, it may seem quite difficult to serve large portions of fish frequently. Moreover, other types of superfoods should also be included in their daily diet for variety in taste and nutrients. It may therefore be necessary to include fish oil supplements in their daily regimen in order to support their growing need for Omega 3.

Chapter 7: Nuts

Nuts are superfoods that should also be included in the dietary requirements of old people. There are a lot of nuts to choose from; so you can give them pistachio, hazelnuts, peanuts, or pecan nuts. But the most nutritious types of nuts are Walnuts and Almonds.

Walnuts

This variety of nuts contains fatty acids, B vitamins, and iron which are all beneficial in maintaining healthy blood cells. The antioxidant property of walnuts is also twice as much as other varieties of nuts, so it is also twice as good.

The omega 3 components of this nut will also provide the elderly with brain power so as to avoid memory loss as they get older. And this fatty acid can also regulate one's cholesterol levels so as to maintain a healthy heart.

In spite of its many benefits, however, walnuts should only be given in moderation. This variety of nuts contains high amounts of calories, so it can result in weight-gain.

Almonds

Aside from being delicious, almonds are rich in copper, riboflavin, and manganese. These are all energy-giving nutrients, so the elderly will particularly benefit from them.

The potassium content of this variety of nuts can also regulate one's blood pressure. The elderly can therefore avoid symptoms of hypertension which is common to their age.

Even respiratory disorders can be avoided through the constant consumption of almonds as it contains antioxidants which can strengthen the lungs. Even one's normal sugar levels can be properly maintained, so it is also good for the diabetic.

The calcium content of almonds will also help in providing the elderly with healthy bones and teeth so that they are more resistant to bone problems (e.g. osteoporosis) and teeth problems (e.g. cavities). Its iron components can also battle symptoms of anemia and dizziness. It even contains vitamin E which helps promote healthy skin and hair.

Almonds are great as snacks. In fact, they are best taken on an empty stomach as their nutrients can be more efficiently absorbed this way.

Benefits of Nuts to the Elderly

A wide variety of nuts can be served regularly to the elderly as this will benefit their overall well-being. As they are filling to the stomach and enjoyable to eat, you won't have any trouble serving these to them.

Antioxidant Properties

The elderly will benefit from the antioxidant properties of nuts because they are at the stage of their lives when their health conditions are extremely fragile. Antioxidants will strengthen their blood vessels to as to avoid any form of inflammation, and they can also defend the body against free radicals that can lead to cancer and other deadly diseases.

High in Fiber

High fiber intake is required of adults as their digestive processes are not as efficient as before. Through the dietary fiber components of nuts, constipation problems can be avoided as regular bowel movement is promoted.

Phytochemical Components

Nuts are rich in phytochemicals too. And these elements prevent the formation of cancer cells inside the body. In fact, they can even destroy existing cancer cells.

Cholesterol Regulator

The Omega 3 component of nuts can help balance the body's good and bad cholesterol. This will help in strengthening the heart of the elderly so that diseases as well as complications can be avoided.

Glucose Regulator

Even those with diabetes can benefit from the food value of nuts. Its potassium content can keep blood sugar levels in its normal rate.

Brain Health

The vitamin E component of nuts can help in maintaining brain health. Memory loss, Alzheimer's disease, and even symptoms of dementia can be delayed or totally avoided.

How Much Nuts Should the Elderly Eat in a Day?

As the condition and dietary requirements of the elderly are different from one another, you should seek the advice of a dietician and a medical practitioner. The amount of nut intake can vary from case to case, but in general, a handful (about 25 grams) a day is safe and beneficial to their health.

Note that nuts should only be given to the elderly as snacks, and not as main meals, as their nutritional value is not high enough. These should also be served long before meal time as they can lose their appetite before a meal.

Chapter 8: Vegetables

Vegetables are natural sources of vitamins, minerals, and antioxidants. These are all needed by the body, and the elderly will especially benefit from them as their health starts to fail them with old age. While all types of vegetables are nutritious, certain groups stand out as superfoods for the elderly. Carrots, broccoli, spinach, tomatoes, kale, and asparagus are among the top veggies that are particularly helpful to old people.

Carrots

Carrot is a versatile crop as it can be used in a lot of different recipes. This can be included in salads, casseroles, soups, and even extracted into juice. While this veggie is particularly popular for its high vitamin A content which aids in eye health, it has other useful components as well.

Beta Carotene

Beta Carotene is one of the many variants of Vitamin A. This is particularly good for the retina as it aids in the cellular health of this particular part of the eye. This makes night vision clear and more efficient for the elderly. And eye diseases like macular degeneration, blindness, and cataracts can also be avoided.

The antioxidant properties of carrots also promote the production of healthy blood cells. And purified blood can help improve the condition of one's skin and hair strands.

The beta carotene component of carrots has also been linked to the prevention of cancer, particularly ovarian and breast cancer. Its healing properties can even improve the deteriorating condition of the lungs in old people.

As one can get overdosed with vitamin A because of its non-water soluble characteristic, its consumption should be monitored closely. A wide variety of vegetables is therefore advised for daily consumption instead of just sticking with one variety.

Vitamin C

There are some Vitamin C components in carrots too; and no matter how small the amount may be, it is still helpful in boosting the body's immune system.

Vitamin C is a well-known antioxidant, so vegetables that carry this nutrient are considered to be anti-aging and anti-cancer as well.

As some of the carrots' vital nutrients can be found on its skin, it is highly recommended that carrots are eaten without peeling off the skin. However, this is only applicable for organic crops as there could be pesticides on the outer layer of the carrots if these are not organic. In this case, it is more advisable to peel off the skin.

Vitamin E

Vitamin E is also an antioxidant that can be linked to anti-aging benefits. It can enhance the brain functions of the elderly so that mental illnesses like Alzheimer's disease, dementia, and even simple memory loss can be avoided or delayed.

This antioxidant also works hand in hand with other vitamins. When combined with vitamins A and C, it can be an effective protection against the damaging effects of the sun's UV rays. In fact, the system also works for effectively for cancer patients who are undergoing radiation therapy and chemotherapy. While cancer cells are killed and destroyed, damaged cellular structures are repaired and rehabilitated.

Zinc

Zinc is also an essential mineral for old people as it helps in the processing of protein and carbohydrates. It also works in enhancing the effects of calcium in the body so that bone problems like osteoporosis can be avoided.

This mineral is also good for the heart, lungs, and prostate. So these organs can remain healthy for a long time. It can even improve the condition of one's hair; so that hair loss, which is associated with aging, can also be kept to a minimum.

Those who are prone to anemia and anorexia will also benefit from the zinc content of carrots as it helps in maintaining the red blood corpuscles healthy and clean. In fact, this mineral can even improve the old folks' sense of taste and smell to stimulate their appetite.

Broccoli

Broccoli is definitely a superfood as its nutritional value is extremely high. It has twice the vitamin C content of oranges, and it is also loaded with antioxidants. This is another one of those versatile ingredients that can be used in a lot of ways in food recipes. So you can serve it steamed, stir-fried, or blanched, or simply include it in vegetable soups and salads. The only thing you need to remember about broccoli is to avoid cooking it in the microwave oven. This process will greatly reduce the amount of nutrients present in the veggie.

Vitamin C

Vitamin C makes the body resistant to flu, colds, and other forms of infection. It also works as an antioxidant in increasing the body's defense against cancer-causing free radicals.

Calcium

The calcium content of broccoli can be better absorbed by the body compared to the calcium content of milk. This can be attributed to the presence of fat in milk which hinders proper absorption of minerals.

Calcium is capable of building and repairing bone structures. It will help the elderly avoid bone problems like osteoporosis and also strengthen their bones against fractures. This mineral is also essential for teeth health so as to avoid chewing problems as one grows old.

Phytonutrients

Phytonutrients are anti-cancer. Regular consumption of broccoli can therefore reduce the risk of developing prostate, breast, pancreatic, and colon cancer among the elderly.

Fiber

Like all other vegetables, broccoli is also loaded with dietary fiber. With enough water intake, this can help reduce constipation problems. Furthermore, fiber also helps maintain proper levels of cholesterol and blood sugar in the body.

Iron

Iron is an essential mineral in the dietary plans of adults as they are prone to blood problems like iron deficiency and anemia. Eating broccoli will provide the elderly with a natural source of iron.

Magnesium

Magnesium benefits the elderly by regulating their blood pressure. Hypertension problems are common to old people, so this mineral should not be missing in their diet.

Selenium

This mineral helps the body combat free radicals. It provides for an overall healthy immune system.

Zinc

The zinc component of broccoli can increase the body's defense system against diseases as it protects the nervous system from being damaged by free radicals. It also helps in oxygenating the brain so as to maintain cognitive awareness even if one gets older and older.

Omega 3 and 6

These are healthy kinds of oil, and they carry anti-inflammatory properties. Both the internal and external organs of the elderly will be efficiently protected by these elements.

Spinach

The superfood spinach is good for the elderly because of its nutritional value. As one of the most popular leafy vegetable, it contains vitamins and minerals which can improve the overall condition of people in their senior years. You can put spinach in soup recipes as well as in sandwiches; and you can also include it in juice concoctions. They can also be served as toppings in lasagna and baked potato recipes.

Flavonoids

This element is a form of antioxidant that will help the body become resistant to cancer. It is particularly effective against oral cavity and lung cancer.

Omega 3 Oil

Omega 3 is a brain booster as it helps in keeping the memory faculty intact and well-functioning even as one ages. Dementia, memory loss, and Alzheimer's disease can be prevented through the regular introduction of this healthy oil to the body.

Vitamin A

The Vitamin A content of spinach will assist the elderly in their vision and skin health. This vitamin is also helpful in keeping the mucous membrane healthy and problem-free.

Protein

Spinach is one of the few veggies that carry high levels of protein. This provides the elderly with energy and it also strengthens the muscles naturally to facilitate effortless body movements.

Vitamin C

As one of the most powerful antioxidants, this vitamin works in strengthening the immune system so that the elderly will not be prone to colds and other infections.

Fiber

Containing high levels of dietary fiber, spinach aids the elderly in their digestion. This reduces the risk of colon cancer as well as other diseases that are caused by poor digestion.

Folate

This element in spinach manages the blood sugar levels to help the elderly avoid deadly complications associated with diabetes.

Lutein

The lutein component in spinach will particularly benefit the eyes. As blindness and macular degeneration have become common to people who are getting old, these ailments can be prevented through this element. In fact, lutein also works against cataracts and cancer.

Tomatoes

While tomatoes technically belong in the fruit family, it is often used as a vegetable ingredient. This type of produce can be used in meal recipes, sauces, salads, soups, and juices. They also serve as nutritious garnishes in sandwich preparations.

Lycopene (Phytochemicals)

One of the major characteristics of phytochemicals is its effectiveness against cancer. It can protect the body's cellular structure from the harmful effects of carcinogenic elements and free radicals in the environment. Cancer of the stomach, pancreas, cervix, colon, breast, and other parts of the human anatomy can therefore be prevented. Lycopene is also helpful in regulating the body's cholesterol levels. This will enable the weakening system of the elderly to become more resistant to heart diseases and other age-related illnesses.

Antioxidants

The antioxidant components present in tomatoes can enhance the body's immunity against infections and diseases due to environmental factors. The effects of UV rays as well as pollution can therefore be minimized and subdued.

Potassium

This mineral is essential for the production of healthy cells in the body. Moreover, it can help in maintaining proper heart rate as well as regulating the body's blood pressure.

Zea-xanthin

This flavonoid compound works in filtering the damaging effects of UV rays to the eyes. It can therefore assist the eye health of the elderly by protecting it against macular degeneration and other similar forms of eye problems.

Vitamin C

As the overall resistance of old people can rapidly decline with the passage of time, a steady source of Vitamin C is extremely needed. This vitamin can strengthen the body's immunity defenses so as to avoid infections and illnesses.

B Complex

B vitamins are important to elderly health because they assist in keeping the nerves and tissues of the body healthy. With enough vitamin B in the system, old people will be less prone to rheumatism and arthritis.

Kale

This variety of green leafy vegetable has a lot of uses as it can be included in soups, casseroles, and even juice recipes. This is easily digestible, that's why it can be easily included in meal plans for the elderly. Moreover it also contains vitamins, minerals, and antioxidants that can help old people cope with the negative effects of aging.

Iron

The iron content of kale assists in the production of healthy red blood cells. This is particularly helpful to old people who are prone to anemia due to iron deficiency.

Calcium

Calcium can strengthen the bones of people in their senior years so that their bones will not easily become brittle and prone to fracture and injury. Osteoporosis, a common illness for aging folks, can also be prevented.

Phytochemicals

The phytochemical components of kale can protect the body from developing cancer diseases like colon and prostate cancer. Furthermore, this element is considered to be an immune system modulator as it can effectively fight viruses and bacteria.

Lutein

Lutein can help maintain healthy eyes in people who are getting old. It also acts as a protector from the sun's ultra violet rays which can be very damaging to the eye's tissues.

Vitamin K

This vitamin is needed by the body to ensure normal blood clotting.

Flavonoids

This antioxidant is anti-inflammatory and anti-cancer as well. It will help old people avoid infections and life-threatening diseases like heart problems and diabetes.

Asparagus

Asparagus can be enjoyed even by picky eaters as its overall taste is pleasant and satisfying. You can serve this to the elderly in steamed or broiled form, or you can simply stir fry them as a side dish. In spite of its delicious taste, this vegetable is loaded with nutrients. That's why it also qualifies as one of the superfoods that can benefit the elderly.

Iron

Sufficient level of iron is essential to old people as they are prone to anemia and other blood problems. By eating asparagus, production of healthy blood cells can be promoted.

Copper

Iron can be better absorbed by the body when there are also copper components in the blood stream. This is also an anti-aging element, so symptoms of old age can be delayed accordingly.

Vitamin K

As this vitamin promotes proper blood clotting, neuronal damages in the brain can be prevented. Alzheimer's disease as well as other mental illnesses can also be avoided.

Fiber

This superfood is high in fiber, so it can regulate cholesterol and blood sugar levels efficiently. As it also aids in proper digestion, constipation problems as well as colon-rectal cancer can be prevented.

Chapter 9: Fruits

Because of the delicious taste of fruits, these can be made into appetizers, desserts, and juices. They can also serve as snacks in their natural form as they are not messy to eat and very satisfying too. Because of their high nutritional value, certain types of fruits are considered to be superfoods. Blueberries, apples, cherries, oranges, and cantaloupe are just some of the most nutritious varieties that can assist the failing health of the elderly.

Blueberries

The elderly will enjoy eating blueberries simply because they're delicious and tasty. This superfood will also benefit their health as it carries high levels of nutrients that will help them in their old age.

Vitamin C

This vitamin is an effective weapon against infections and different kinds of complications. It will therefore benefit old people a lot as their resistance against various diseases is increased.

Antioxidants

The antioxidant properties found in blueberries far outweigh the antioxidant contents of other fruits and vegetables. This provides the body with power to combat the daily exposure to free radicals.

Dietary Fiber

As blueberries are loaded with fiber, symptoms of constipation and other stomach problems can be avoided. Furthermore, it also makes the body resistant to debilitating diseases like cancer of the colon.

Flavonoid

This compound can help the failing health of old folks by limiting the effects of free radicals that can lead to heart problems and cancer.

Vitamin B

B vitamins can help strengthen the body's nerves and boost brain activity too. Cognitive impairment, which is common to the elderly, can be delayed by up to 2 and a half years.

Apples

Apples make for a great snack and they can be easily appreciated even by people in their old age. The nutritional value of apples has always been documented as one of the best, that's why it is considered to be one of the strongest superfoods around.

Vitamin C

Recent studies have revealed that apples contain just as much vitamin C as oranges, if not more. This makes the fruit a powerful defense against bodily infections and deadly diseases.

Phytonutrients

Phytochemical compounds make a certain fruit or vegetable anti-cancer. Aside from preventing the multiplication of cancer cells, even the existing ones can be killed and destroyed once the level of phytonutrients in the body is increased.

Flavonoids

This antioxidant works in battling free radicals. So it can help strengthen the overall health of the elderly.

Potassium

The potassium content of apples can improve the condition of the body's nervous system. It makes old people less susceptible to arthritis and rheumatism.

Cherries

Cherries can be eaten as snacks or included in desserts, salads and juices. Its high nutritional content qualifies it to be labeled as a superfood as even the elderly can become stronger through the constant consumption of this fruit.

Iron

This fruit is high in iron, so it can assist in the proper production of red blood corpuscles. Those with blood problems, particularly anemia, can benefit from this mineral.

Flavonoid

This antioxidant compound can increase the body's resistance against life threatening diseases like cancer.

Melatonin

This element can provide the brain with soothing effects. A person's mood and irritability can therefore be regulated so as not to cause any kind of stress. It can even help remove symptoms of headaches and insomnia. And as old folks tend to suffer from depression and anxiety, regular intake of this element is advised in order to improve one's condition.

Potassium

As potassium is good for the nerves, cramps, joint pains, and muscle spasms can be reduced. This mineral also benefits the heart as it works in regulating the body's blood pressure.

Zinc

This element assists the proper absorption of calcium in order to aid in bone health. It can also strengthen the lungs so as to avoid respiratory illnesses like pneumonia and cancer.

Oranges

The elderly should definitely eat oranges in order to supply the body with high amounts of natural vitamin C. Because of its pleasant taste, it can be served as snacks or as juices.

Antioxidants

The antioxidant properties of oranges can help cleanse and strengthen the body. It can also delay the signs of aging by improving the condition of the hair and skin.

Pectin

This component works in protecting the mucous membrane so as to decrease its exposure to toxic elements. By binding itself to cancer-causing substances in the digestive system, colon cancer can be avoided. Pectin also helps in lowering the body's bad cholesterol levels.

Vitamin C

This is a popular component in oranges. In fact, oranges are said to be the highest carriers of vitamin C. This vitamin is needed by the elderly as it helps in increasing the body's resistance against germs and viruses.

Vitamin A

Vitamin A can also be found in oranges; and this aids in keeping the eyes, skin, and mucous membranes healthy. It can also slow down the degenerative effects of aging.

Flavonoids

The flavonoid compounds contained in oranges serve as antioxidants that can deter the occurrence of cancer. By strengthening the body's resistance, old people will become less prone to debilitating diseases.

Vitamin B

B vitamins can help lessen nerve problems in old people. By keeping the muscles, tissues and nerve endings pliable, one will be less prone to joint pains as well as muscle pains.

Calcium

The elderly need a large amount of calcium in their body as their bone and teeth health start to deteriorate rapidly. Problems like osteoporosis and loss of teeth can be avoided through the provision of this mineral.

Cantaloupe

The sweet taste of cantaloupe makes it ideal as desserts or snacks. This can be regularly served to the elderly as they are loaded with vitamins and minerals that can help the body cope up with the problems of getting old.

Vitamin C

Aside from boosting the body's immune system, this vitamin also works as an antioxidant. It aids in keeping the mucous membrane, eyes, and skin healthy.

Vitamin A

This vitamin is also an antioxidant, and it helps in making the body resistant to lung and oral cavity diseases.

Potassium

As this mineral can strengthen the heart and properly regulate the body's blood pressure, diseases like coronary heart disease and stroke can be avoided.

Carotenoids

The carotenoid component of cantaloupe can assist in eye health. Vision loss, cataract, glaucoma and other eye diseases can be prevented through this element.

Magnesium

This element is important in an old person's diet as it can provide the body with energy. Moreover, it also helps in regulating the body's temperature so as not to become vulnerable to cold weather.

Folate

Folate helps in producing healthy red blood corpuscles in order to avoid symptoms of anemia. This element is also an anti-cancer agent.

Fiber

As this fruit is rich in dietary fiber, it can promote regular bowel movement. Constipation problems can also be avoided accordingly.

Chapter 10: Dairy

Not all dairy products are good for old people because some varieties may carry too many calories that can lead to an increase in weight and other complications. Furthermore, certain dairy products can also increase one's cholesterol levels which can be particularly dangerous to the elderly because they are more prone to heart attacks than younger people. Yogurt and low-fat milk are 2 kinds of dairy products that can benefit people over the age of 50. In spite of belonging to the low-calorie food group, they contain vitamins, minerals, and good bacteria that allow them to be labeled as superfoods.

Yogurt

Yogurt has always been recommended for weight-loss programs and other dietary plans. Its high nutritional value and positive effects on the digestive system enable the body to become more resistant to infectious diseases. This can be taken as desserts or snacks, and you will not find it hard to serve this to the elderly as they can surely appreciate its taste and overall effects to their health.

Calcium

As the main source of yogurt is milk, it also carries high amounts of calcium. This mineral is essential for bone health so that fractures and diseases like osteoporosis can be prevented. Moreover, it also promotes healthy teeth so as not to have chewing problems.

Probiotics

The probiotics contained in yogurt assist in proper digestion of food and bowel regularity. This is especially helpful to old people as their digestive system is no longer as efficient as before.

B2 Vitamin

The presence of B2 in the body can help the system in coping with stress and fatigue.

B12

B12 stimulates the production of healthy red blood cells. Aside from the prevention of anemia, it also aids in the proper circulation of oxygen in the entire body.

Potassium

The potassium content of yogurt helps in maintaining the right level of blood pressure, so that symptoms of hypertension can be avoided.

Low-Fat Milk

The elderly are strongly advised to drink milk regularly because of its nutritional contents. However, not all types of milk are considered to be good, as they can contain fat and calories. Because of the sensitive condition of old people, only low-fat milk is recommended in order to avoid cholesterol build-up. With the low-fat variety, one can still get the benefits of the milk product without endangering the health.

Calcium

Milk is one of the main sources of calcium. This mineral is needed by people who are growing old as the bone in their bodies start to weaken and deteriorate. Calcium can strengthen the bones again, and ailments like osteoporosis can also be avoided through proper nourishment of this mineral.

Protein

The protein content of milk can prevent the deterioration of muscle mass. It also provides the body with energy so that one will not feel lethargic and weak.

Phosphorous

This is another mineral that aids in bone health. It makes the bones and teeth healthier and stronger.

Vitamin A

This vitamin is an anti-aging component in milk. It helps one get smoother and more pliable skin, so that the appearance of wrinkles and lines can be minimized.

Chapter 11: Grain

There are also grain products that can be considered as superfoods because of their nutritional value and cleansing effects to the system. Oats are recommended to the elderly because they can aid in proper digestion and provide the body with nutritional elements too.

Oats

Oats can be consumed in various forms. When served as oatmeal, these can be eaten as porridge. Other products of oats include oat breads and oatmeal cookies; and there are also oat cakes. Oatmeal is commonly eaten at breakfast or during snack time. Old people will not have a problem eating porridge as these are soft-textured and easy on the teeth and stomach. You can add variety to oatmeal by adding fruits and honey to the mixture. This way, the meal will become even more nutritious and delectable.

Fiber

The fiber content of oats is extremely high, so it greatly helps in digestion as well as in lowering the body's cholesterol levels. Regular intake of high-fiber foods will lessen constipation issues as well as heart problems.

Calcium

Oats contain some calcium components that will assist the body in avoiding bone and dental problems.

Zinc

This mineral helps the body to recover from illnesses faster. It also facilitates fast healing of wounds.

Iron

The iron content of oats helps in minimizing blood problems that can lead to anemia.

Chapter 12: Healthy Beverages

There are certain beverages that are considered to be superfoods because of their overall effects to the human body. Because of the sensitive condition of the elderly, only the right types of beverages should be served to them. Some of the safe and nutritional drinks that can be given to them include green tea, black tea, and red wine.

Green Tea

Green teas have always been known for their many health benefits and low-caffeine content. This makes for a great alternative to coffees as too much caffeine can be dangerous to old people with heart problems.

Antioxidants

The high amount of antioxidants present in green tea allows for the eradication of free radicals in the system.

Furthermore, complications that can result in the frail conditions of the elderly can be avoided as the body is made to be stronger and more resistant to diseases.

Anti-Aging

Green tea also carries anti-aging properties that can slow down the natural deterioration of the body. It can prevent the early onset of memory loss and even improve one's overall appearance.

Soothing Effects

Another health benefit of drinking green tea is its soothing and calming effects. Because of this, old people will not be as prone to depression, restlessness and insomnia.

Black Tea

Black tea is another variety of drink that's healthy and beneficial to the elderly. However, this type of tea has more caffeine content than green tea, so it should be given in moderation to people who are sensitive to caffeine or to those that have ulcer problems. You can also get the decaffeinated types to still benefit from the drink without being affected by the caffeine.

Antioxidants

This is another type of tea that's loaded with antioxidant properties. These compounds can effectively battle free radicals so that there will be minimal damage to the body's DNA composition. It also allows the body to recuperate faster when there are infections or inflammations.

For Cardiovascular Health

Because of the heart-friendly elements present in black tea, the risk of suffering from strokes can be prevented. This is especially true for the decaffeinated variety, as caffeine can sometimes cause palpitations.

Diabetes-Friendly

Sugar-free black tea can be served to those who have diabetes. It contains antioxidant compounds that can regulate the blood sugar levels inside the body efficiently.

For Mental Clarity

The natural ingredients in black tea enable proper oxygenation of the brain. One's mental state can therefore be enhanced, and mental ailments like Alzheimer's disease and Parkinson's disease can also be avoided.

Red Wine

A glass of red wine in a day can benefit even the elderly. This type of drink carries certain compounds that can enhance the overall health of people who are getting old.

Bioflavonoids

The antioxidants contained in red wine can help prevent blood clotting and strokes.

Resveratrol

This component allows the body to maintain a healthy level of cholesterol, so that coronary problems can be avoided.

Tannins

This element strengthens the veins and arteries of the heart so as to lessen the impact of saturated fats.

Alcohol

The small dosage of alcohol content in red wine can increase the good cholesterol in the body.

Polyphenols

This compound aids in oral health as it helps in avoiding gum problems.

Antioxidants

The antioxidant properties of red wine can delay the signs of aging (sagging skin, wrinkles, memory loss, etc.). These same compounds can also help prevent degenerative diseases like cancer, Alzheimer's disease, and diabetes.

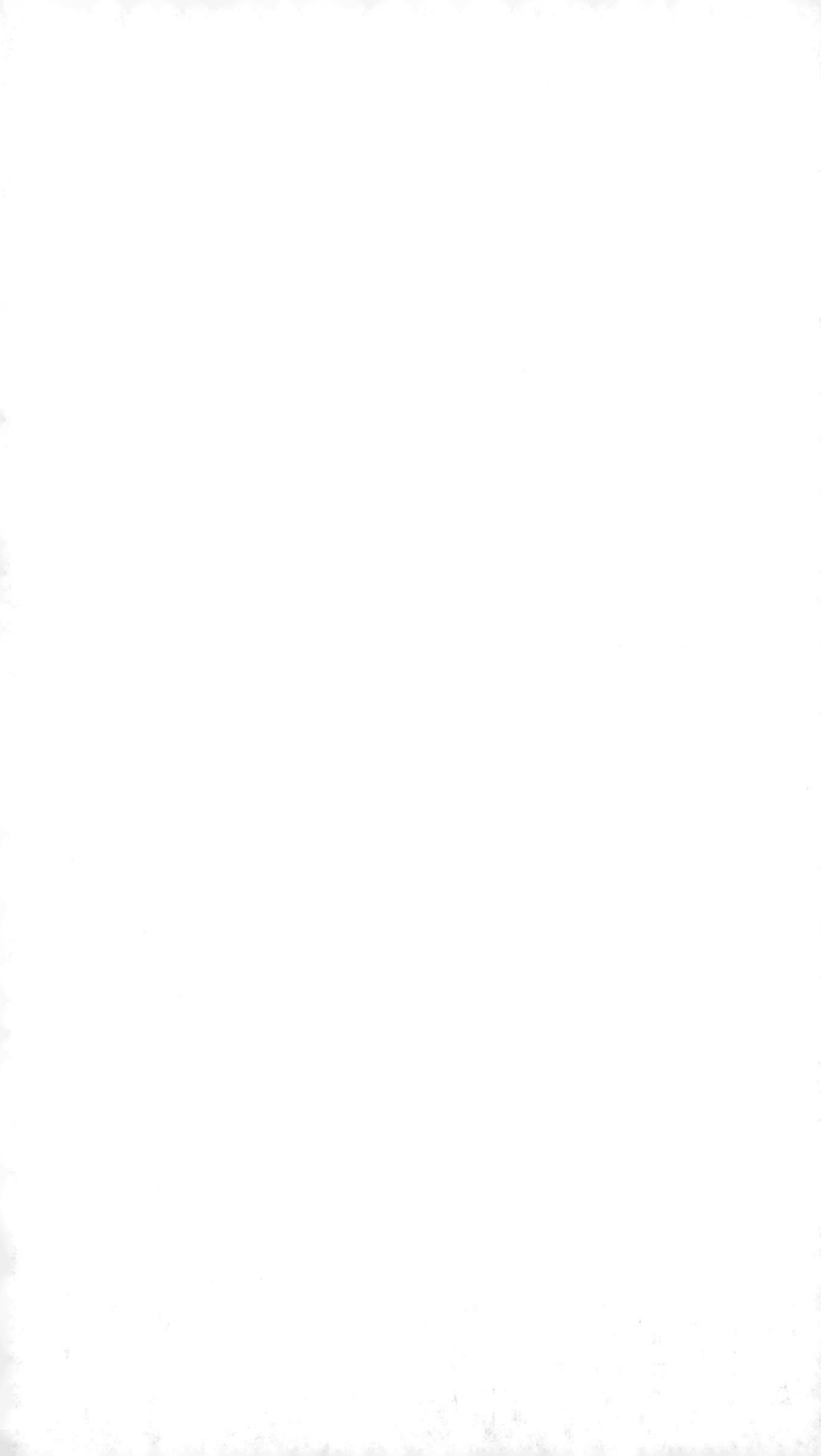

www.ingramcontent.com/pod-product-compliance
Lightning Source LLC
Chambersburg PA
CBHW060643290526
45793CB00001B/382